The Karezza Method

Magnetation, The Art of Connubial Love

By John William Lloyd

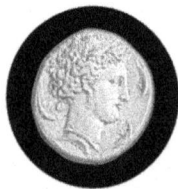

PANTIANOS
CLASSICS

Published by Pantianos Classics

ISBN-13: 978-1-78987-214-9

First published in 1931

Contents

Preface

It was, I believe, in the winter of 1915-16 that a woman-friend in California wrote and asked me why I did not write a special little book on Karezza.

As events had convinced me that there certainly was crying need of instruction on the matter, her suggestion took root and this small brochure is the fruit.

For though quite a number have written more or less concerning controlled intercourse, they have usually done so guardedly and so vaguely that to the average inquirer the subject remains a mystery and the beginner does not know how to proceed. For which reason most men fail and give up who could just as well succeed. And success or failure here may make all the difference between divorce or a lifetime of love-happiness.

Soul-Blending

And still beyond the embrace that begets the body is the embrace that begets the soul, that invokes the soul from the Soul.

The wonderful embraces, sacred, occult and unspeakably tender, pure as prayer;

The hour-long, longer indwelling of him within her, conceiving her again like a child, the hour-long, longer, over-closing of her upon him, bearing him again like a babe in her womb.

The infinite understanding of each by the other, the transcendent uplift of each by the other;

No tumult orgasmal here; not because crushed out, simply because not desired, simply because this is beyond that, a saner, broader joy; the great currents, flowing through wider channels, rage not nor whirl, for where the greater is there the lesser is not demonstrative.

Here is harmony too sweet for violence, osmosis of soul within soul, rhythmically blending, inflowing, outflowing; singing without words; silent music of divine instrument.

Symphony of sex of nerve, heart, thought, and soul in touch, at-one-ing.

Absolute peace, realized heaven, the joy that never disappoints, that exceeds imagination, that cannot be described.

The love ineffable, the inspiration of brain, the energizing of muscle, the illumination of feature, the healing of body, the expression of soul.

Spiritual sex-exchanging; the masculine in her uttering, the feminine in him receiving, positive and negative alternating at will.

Spiritual sex-begetting; the impregnation of each by the other with beautiful thoughts, divine dreams, high hopes, noble ambitions, pure aspirations, clairvoyant vision, the birth-bed of genius.

The giving of each to the other to the uttermost impulse of blessing, the receiving of each by the other to the uttermost nerve terminal of body, to the uttermost fine filament of spirit.

Not followed by exhaustion, but by days of genius, clear and exalted vision, buoyant and happy health.

Not followed by revulsion, but by hours, days, weeks, years, a lifetime, maybe, of tender memories, clinging, affectionate longing to caress again, to be re-embracing.

(Nay, is it not true, beyond all truth, that those who have once thus bathed, blended, soul in soul, are eternally married?)

The embrace of at-one-ness, of expression, and purification and revivification, that incarnates the divine in the human.

Not possible except to the pure and poetic, to true and innocent lovers, fitting, responding, liberating.

To whom soul and body are both sacred, to whom this communion is a religious rite the most sacred.

The embrace of the Cosmic souls, the angel-mates in their heaven.

No vision this, dear friends, no poetic metaphor merely, for lo! I have lived it all many, many times, hundreds of others have lived it many times, every member of the race shall sometime, in some life, live it.

It is joy and truth, the joy of joys and truth of truths. KAREZZA

It is my hope that in this work I shall be able to give the world a plain, practical little guidebook to what I consider the most important sexual discovery and practice in all human history.

What Is Karezza?

Karezza is controlled non-seminal intercourse. The word Karezza (pronounced Ka-ret-za) is from the Italian and means a caress. Alice B. Stockham, M.D., was the first one who applied it as the distinctive name of the art and method of sexual relations without orgasmal conclusion. But the art and method itself was discovered in 1844 by John Humphrey Noyes, the founder of the Oneida Community, by experiences and experiments in his own marital life. He called it Male Continence. Afterwards George N. Miller, a member of the Community, gave it the name of Zugassent's Discovery in a work of fiction, *The Strike of a Sex*. There are objections to both these names. Zugassent was not a real person, therefore did not discover it. It was Noyes' Discovery, in fact. Continence, as Dr. Stockham points out, has come to mean abstinence from all intercourse. The Oneida Communists do not appear to have opposed the female orgasm, therefore it was well enough for them to name it Male Continence, but Dr. Stockham and I agree that in the highest form and best expression of the art neither man nor, woman has or desires to have the orgasm, therefore it is no more male than female continence. And a single-word name is always more convenient than a compound. For which reasons I have accepted Dr. Stockham's musical term, which is besides, beautifully suggestive and descriptive. Another writer on this art (I first heard of it through him; he deriving it from Noyes) was Albert Chavannes, who in a little book on it, called it Magnetation, a name which I coined for him. It is perhaps not a bad name; but I now think Karezza better.

Noyes' honor to the discovery has been disputed. Others, it is asserted, discovered it before him or independently since. [1] It is necessary to contest this. Various Europeans and Asiatics probably discovered America before Columbus, but he first made it known and helpful to the world at large, therefore the honor is rightfully his. Exactly so with Noyes - he first made Karezza available to mankind in general.

His little work, *Male Continence*, is a model of good argument on the matter; but I believe *Karezza*, by Dr. Stockham, is the only book now in print which treats of it. Several other small works have appeared, but mostly they treat of the subject in such poetic and transcendental terms that the seeker after practical instruction is left still seeking. All writers, too, have tacitly assumed that the woman could do as she pleased in the matter and that success or failure all depended on the man. I regard this as a fundamental error and the cause of most disappointments. Considerations such as these have mainly decided me to write this little work. At this time of agitation on birth control, also, it appears timely. And beyond all looms the extraordinary, one might say unaccountable ignorance of it, not only of ordinary sexual students, but of practically all physicians and even the greatest sexual specialists and teachers. Actually the general public knows more about it than its educators. Thus Forel, in his *Sexual Question*, never mentions it at all, therefore presumably never heard of it. Bloch, in his professedly exhaustive work, *The Sexual Life of Our Times*, though he once mentions Dr. Stockham on another matter, has only one ambiguous paragraph in the whole book that can possibly refer to Karezza (apparently some imperfect form of it), disapproving of it on theory only, evidently, without the slightest personal knowledge, or even observation. Havelock Ellis, in the *Psychology of Sex*, is more instructed and favorable, but appears to have derived his knowledge almost entirely from the Oneida Communists; not at all at first hand. And the general ignorance, indifference, or aversion, even to any experiment, among men, is simply amazing. Most men say at once that it is impossible, most physicians that it is injurious, though with no kind of real knowledge. Most women, on the other hand, who have had any experience of it, eulogize it in unmeasured terms, as the very salvation of their sexual life, the very art and poetry of love, which indeed it is, but, as most men will not attempt it, most women are necessarily kept in ignorance of its inestimable benefits to their sex.

The first objection that is certain to meet one who would recommend Karezza is that it is "unnatural." Noyes confronts this objection very ably, and it is indeed absurd, when you came to think of it, to hear men who drink alcohol, smoke, use tea and coffee, take milk, though adults, eat cooked food, live in heated houses, wear clothes, write books, shave their faces, use machinery, and do a thousand and one things which the natural man, the true aborigine, knew nothing of, condemn a mere act of moderation and self-control in pleasure as "unnatural."

They do not stop to think that if their appeal is to original or animal nature, then they must never have intercourse with the female at all, except when she invites it, is in a certain condition, at certain seasons of the year, and for procreation only. For all intercourse as a love act is clearly "unnatural" in their use of the term. How would they relish that?

These same men will recommend and have their women use douches, drugs, and all sorts of mechanical means to nullify the natural consequences of their act, with never a lisp of protest at the unnaturalness of it all.

As a matter of fact, Karezza is absolutely natural. It employs Nature only and from first to last. To check any act which prudence suggests, or experience has shown, likely to have undesired consequences, is something constantly done throughout all Nature, even among the lowest animals. Karezza is such a check. It is simply prudence and skill in the sexual realm, changing its form and direction of activity in such wise that the desired pleasure may be more fully realized and the undesired results avoided. Nothing more.

The denunciation of it as injurious is almost equally an expression of thoughtless prejudice. I have now had personal knowledge of it for over forty years. I learned of it from A. Chavannes, who with his wife had practiced it twenty years. It has been before the American people since 1846. The Oneida Communists practiced it, Havelock Ellis states, thirty years. I have known members of the Oneida Community. I have read all I possibly could on it, talked with everyone I could hear of who had knowledge of it; I have yet to meet or hear of a single woman who has the slightest accusation to make against it on the score of injury to health or disagreeable sensations or after effects. Three only (all with slight experience) told me they thought there was more pleasure in the old embrace; the others most emphatically to the contrary. Van de Warker, says, Havelock Ellis, "studied forty-two women of the community without finding any undue prevalence of reproductive diseases, *nor could he find any diseased condition attributable to the sexual habits of the community.*" (Italics mine.) Contrast this with the usual sex-relation, which is constantly being accused, particularly by women, of causing all sorts of injurious and painful consequences, apparently upon the best of evidence. After twenty-five years experience, the Oneida Community, upon request of the New York *Medical Gazette*, instituted "a professional examination" and had a report made by Theodore R. Noyes, M.D., in which it was shown, by careful comparison of our statistics with those of the U. S. census and other public documents, that the rate of nervous diseases in the Community is considerably below the average of ordinary society. This report was published by the *Medical Gazette*, and was pronounced by the editor "a model of careful observation; bearing intrinsic evidence of entire honesty and impartiality."

Physicians freely condemn it, or express doubts of it, almost invariably with no knowledge of it of any kind. They think it *should* cause ill-health, therefore they say it *will*. It is said to cause nervousness, prostatitis, an inflamed state of organs, etc. Now we all know how much pure guesswork figures in so-called medical "science"; how often that which merely coincides is asserted to hold a relation of cause and effect. However I think I can see how, very easily, the ignorant or imperfect use of this art might lead to the above-described bad results. In ideal and successful Karezza the sexual passion is transmuted and sublimated, to a greater or less degree, into tenderness and love, and the thought is maintained that the orgasm is not desired or desirable. Now if a man, on the contrary, entered the embrace with the thought that he terribly desired the orgasm, but by the sheer force of will must prevent it; if he excited himself and his partner to the utmost sexual furore, but at last denied it culmination; caring nothing for love at any time, but for sex only all the time, I can see how, very reasonably, his denied passion might react disastrously on his nervous system, just as any strongly repressed emotion may. Just as a man who indulges in the most furious thoughts of rage, but clenches his fists and shuts his mouth tight, rather than express it, may burst a blood vessel or get an apoplexy. This may indeed be a sort of "male continence," on the physical side, but real Karezza, as I know it and would present it, is very different.

Real Karezza requires preparatory mental exercise. It requires first the understanding and conviction that the spiritual, the caressive, the tender side of the relation is much more important, much more productive of pleasure in fact, than the merely sexual, and that throughout the whole relation the sexual is to be held subordinate to this love side as its tool, its agent, its feeder. Sex is indeed required to furnish all it has to the feast, but strictly under the leadership of and to the glory of love.

It requires, second, the understanding and profound conviction that in this kind of love-feast the orgasm is a marplot, a kill-joy, an awkward and clumsy accident, and the end of everything for the time, therefore most undesired.

It requires, third, an understanding of the psychological law that all emotions are to a considerable extent capable of being "sublimated," that is expressed in a different direction and with reference to another object than that first intended. We have all seen orators or actors first arouse an audience to emotional intensity and then direct that emotion at pleasure to laughter or tears, to love or hate, revenge or pity, lust or purity. Taking full advantage of this law, the Karezza artist sublimates a portion of his sexual passion into the more refined, intellectual, poetic and heart-sweet expression of feeling, thus preventing it from ever reaching that pitch of local intensity which demands explosive discharge. In other words the soul, taking over the blind sex-emotion, diffuses it and irradiates the whole being for a prolonged period with its joy-giving, exalting potency. This might be compared to a man who had a barrel of gunpowder where with to celebrate, whereupon instead of firing the entire cask in one mighty explosion (orgasm) he made it into fire-works for the esthetic enjoyment of a whole evening. Observe that either way all the powder would be burned, only in the second form the display covers a much greater length of time, is more refined, artistic and complexly satisfying.

Such is Karezza to the orgasm. It is art, intellect, morality and estheticism in sexual enjoyment instead of crude, reckless appetite.

Still this comparison does not do Karezza justice. When the powder is burned it is gone, but it is not at all so with Karezza. In Nature something accumulates in the organism for the endowment of the offspring. Much of man's food consists of what lower forms of life have stored up for their children - we largely live on starch, honey, gluten, seeds, milk, eggs, robbed from babies that were to be. In our own bodies also we store up a reproductive surplus to be given to our progeny. This is probably not simply one thing, but many things - love, magnetism, vital force, seed, perhaps other things that we know nothing about today, and indeed we do not know very accurately about any of these things today, but we do know that *something* is stored up in us, and that its presence in us makes us vivid, brilliant, beautiful, powerful, like a stimulating food. It is a life-food or life-force, intended to be given to our children, but we also can feed on it or give it to each other. Love between a man and woman seems to be such a process of mutually exchanging and feeding on this surplus life-force. When they enter each other's aura there is an interchange of male and female food-values; the nearer they are to each other the stronger and more satisfying the exchange, and their "love" to each other is the craving for such an exchange or the thing itself, hence the craving for *closeness*and *touch*. In Karezza, both by reason of its intense intimacy and of the long time of contact, besides the peculiar fitness of the organs themselves for the work, this exchange reaches its maximum of realization - it is vital exchange in its most satisfying expression - wherefore it is really the thing for which all love is reaching, wishing.

Apparently, in the love-contact of two, some of this life-food is released in each and reabsorbed in each, but more of it is given to the other partner. Men and women in love are thus veritable cannibals and feed each on each, and each gives to the other the stored-up life-food, charged with the personal qualities of maleness or femaleness of the individual sex. Apparently my lover and I may live on our life-foods to some extent, but each finds the life-food of the other the more stimulating and nutritious. In Karezza we feed each other "baby food."

Explain the process as we may, this fact is sure, that in successful Karezza the sex-organs become quiet, satisfied, demagnetized, as perfectly as by the orgasm, while the rest of the body of each partner glows with a wonderful vigor and conscious joy, or else with a deep, sweet, contentment, as after a happy play; tending to irradiate the whole being with romantic love; and always with an after-feeling of health, purity and wellbeing. We are most happy and good-humored as after a full meal. Whereas, if there has been an orgasm, it is the common experience that there is a sense of loss, weakness, and dispelled illusion; following quickly on the first grateful feeling of relief. There has been a momentary joy, but too brief and epileptic to make much impression on consciousness, and now it is gone, leaving no memory. The lights have gone out, the music has stopped. The weakness is often so severe as to cause pallor, faintness, vertigo, dyspepsia, disgust, irritability, shame, dislike, or other pathological or unloving symptoms. This especially on the man's part, but perhaps to some extent on the woman's part too. Even if no more, there is lassitude, sudden indifference, a wish to sleep. A wet blanket has fallen for the time at least, on the flame of love. Romance drops and crawls like a winged bird.

In Karezza, on, the contrary, the partners unfold and separate reluctantly, lingeringly, kissing, clinging, petting to the last, thrilled with and rehearsing memories, glowing with an affection and admiration which they feel can never end.

It would appear that in the orgasmal embrace the life-force is thrown off with such suddenness and volume that it is quite impossible for the partner to receive or assimilate much of it, therefore most of it is utterly wasted.

For this reason, the orgasmal-embrace is a most clumsy and disappointing thing when employed as a love-embrace. Nature meant it only for propagation and its whole *modus operandi* is calculated to check love, defeat love, and turn love into indifference or aversion. The more frequently it is employed, the more love dies, romance evaporates, and a mere sexuality, a matter-of-fact relation, or plain dislike, takes the place of the glamour of courtship days. On the contrary, Karezza makes marriage more delicious than courtship, more romantic than wooing, and maintains an endless, satisfying honeymoon.

There is an increase of attractiveness and magnetism of each for each, a growth of satisfaction in each other's society, affection, and caressing becomes a sweet habit.

Nothing else known makes the course of true love run so smooth as Karezza.

The orgasm is not always, but very commonly followed by a greater or less degree of exhaustion, perhaps extreme, but Karezza, unless repeated to excess, or practiced between the mismated, is *never* followed by exhaustion, but often by a delightful glow and joy in life. The usual sequel to the orgasm is demagnetization, indifference, too frequently irritability, disgust, repulsion and a craving for stimulants, but Karezza irradiates the whole being with tender, romantic, peaceful love. This, so far as I know, is universal experience, therefore merely needs to be stated to show how healthful an influence Karezza must wield. As a matter of fact, because of the tonicity, glow and vigor it bestows on the sexual parts and its wine-like inspiration of the spirit of the partners, with no reaction, it is one of the best hygienic agencies for the benefit and cure of ordinary sexual weaknesses and ailments - leucorrhea, displacements, prolapsus, bladder-troubles, simple urethritis, prostatitis, [2] etc., known. And I say this from actual knowledge. I have known it to act like magic in painful menstruation and in prostatitis. But remember, I am always speaking of its exercise between those who are naturally fitted to respond and who really love each other, who honor their bodies and would not knowingly abuse them. As a mere sex-experiment it might be of little value or satisfaction. It appears to be perfect or poor, just about in proportion to the greater or less amount of heart-love involved. At least it imperatively demands kindness, tenderness, chivalry on the man's part, a pleased acceptance and relaxation on the woman's; and the more refinement, poetry of feeling and mutual romance the better - any amount can be utilized. The gross, reckless and lustful may as well let it alone - it is not for them.

As a nerve sedative its effect is remarkable. I have known it to instantly cure a violent, even agonizing nervous headache, a restful nap following upon the cessation of pain. Under a strong, gentle magnetic man, a nervous woman often falls into a baby-like sleep, in the very midst of the embrace, and this is felt to be a peculiar luxury and coveted experience. Many women call Karezza "The Peace"; others call it "Heaven." This alone is a testimony worth volumes.

S. G. Lewis, of Grass Valley, California, in his *Hints and Keys to Conjugal Felicity*, is especially rich in testimony to the spiritual and romantic value of Karezza, but his fine little work is long out of print.

Now I do not apprehend, from all I have seen of life, that Karezza will ever come into vogue from the male side of the world. Men seem united in their dull, lethargic indifference to it. Helplessly or selfishly they say it is impossible, and let it go at that, rather than make the little effort required to perfect themselves in it. They would preferably choose, or rather oblige their women to choose, something out of the nerve-shocking, disgusting, disease-producing outfit of douches, drugs, tampons, plugs, pessaries, shields, condoms, and save them all further responsibility in the matter, although the highest authorities admit none of these resources are really safe, that is sure, contraceptives, and most of them are decidedly injurious. *Only the absence of semen is safe*, and that is found in Karezza and in Karezza alone. But perhaps the most clinching condemnation of these methods, to a refined person, is that pronounced by a fine woman of my acquaintance, "There is not one of these methods that does not destroy, *for the woman*, all the poetry of the act." Only in Karezza is the poetry fully preserved, and not only that, but made capable of development to the most refined nuances of artistic and ingenious delight. Only to the Karezza-lover is the Art of Love possible in any sense worthy of the name. All the others begin the performance by shutting off the music and throwing away the wine.

But as the Woman Movement grows I am sure Karezza will come into its own. As women learn its transcendent importance to their happiness and health, they will demand it and refuse all men that cannot supply that demand. That will be a force that cannot be withstood.

Woman is by birth the Queen of Love and will certainly assume her inheritance and control in her own sphere and realm.

[1] Since writing the above I have become acquainted with a Dr. E. Elmer Keeler, of Syracuse, New York, who tells me that he made the independent discovery of Karezza, by his own sex-experiences in early manhood, and for years taught it in private lectures, both to the laity and the profession, before he learned of Noyes and his teaching — a sufficient commentary, if any were needed, on the ig-

norance not only of the general public, but even of the doctors, on this most important matter. Not knowing of any other, Keeler gave it the name of "Sex-communion," but defining the term as "ALL forms of sexual expression in which no emission occur," thus still leaving a need for a specific term to name the definite internal act, which Karezza as a term does.

[2] [Leucorrhea is vaginal discharge, prolapsus is the slipping of the uterus, urethritis is inflammation of the urethra, and prostatitis is inflammation of the prostate gland.]

Magnetation

As I have said, I coined for Albert Chavannes, as a title for his little brochure on this subject, the word "Magnetation." This was intended to express the theory, then so prevalent, that the thrills and pleasures of sex and love were caused by the transmission and reception of currents of "animal magnetism," or "vital electricity," which could be conveyed by contact or passes from one human body to another, and that diseases even could be cured by the same agency, as in "laying on of hands." There has been much controversy on this matter. It has been argued by some that the "currents," the "magnetic attractions," etc., felt by the susceptible, were purely imaginary and ideological, - that the lover induced his own thrills, the patient cured himself. We may waive much of this. While today one hears very little of this magnetism, the fact remains that the presence and the touch, explain it as we may, of certain people, give us intense, vivid feelings and produce powerful reactions, while the presence and touch of others may shock, or leave us indifferent or repelled. Practically this is sufficient. This seems like magnetic action and for all our purposes we may assume that the seeming is a fact.

It is assumed therefore that ordinarily the male is positive to the female, who is negative to him, and the masculine organs are positive to the feminine organs. This may be called the normal or usual relation, but it is possible to voluntarily or involuntarily reverse this, and in most cases, between lovers in close contact, certain parts in each are negative to the contacting parts of the other, which may be positive to them. This fact, that the entire personality, in all its parts, is not necessarily positive or negative at the same time, is one important to remember, for it explains much and is like a key to the whole art of Karezza. Thus a woman may be very positive and even dominant in her love, while her body remains most alluringly passive. Or she may open her eyes and make them positive while the rest remains negative. Or she may put positiveness into the caress of her hands alone, or will it into some other part of her being, or entirely assume and play the masculine, positive part, while the man assumes the feminine. Of this more will be said later.

But in general, though the woman allures and makes herself a drawing lodestone, it is the man who takes and should take the active, positive role and is "the artist in touch." The man who would succeed in Karezza, then, must cultivate the art of magnetic touch. He should learn to think of himself as an electric battery, of which it may be said that the right hand is the positive pole (in right-handed people only, of course), and the left hand the negative, capable of transmitting to other and receptive human beings an electric current. If both his hands are in contact with someone, he must feel the current flowing from his right hand *through* the body he touches into his left hand, and he must learn how to reverse this and send a current at will *from* his left hand *to* his right hand. If he touches with only one hand, or one part, then he must feel that he touches positively and the flesh he touches is negative or receptive to him. He must learn to will the current he gives through the body he touches, through its nerves, to any part he wishes to electrify, to thrill or to soothe, and to feel convincingly that he is doing so. In Karezza his organs must ordinarily be felt to be positive, and the woman's negative, for the best results to both. He may even practice on himself, learning to feel his own magnetism, to test it; and how to cure various pains and ailments by his own touch.

Understand me - a man may succeed beautifully in Karezza who has done nothing of all this, nor even heard of it, because of natural magnetism and intuition of what to do, but even he would do better to consciously understand his powers and deliberately will to direct their use.

The fact that magnetic touch has been found a successful method of invigorating the weak and curing the sick, is one proof that should never be overlooked that Karezza, practiced normally, with a wise avoidance of excess, is not only not injurious, as so often claimed, but is really conducive to health. I have been told that Harry Gaze, the Western lecturer, advocates Karezza as a means of maintaining eternal youth, and personally I am convinced that nothing else known is so efficient in preserving youth, hope, beauty, romance and the joy of life.

A man should learn, therefore, to touch the woman he loves in such a way that he transmits to her a vivid electric current that thrills her with delightful feeling, while it relieves his nervous tension of accumulated surplus force. At the same time, if the parties are well-mated, she will be generating and returning, in some roundabout way, something to him, which equally satisfies him, prevents all sense of loss, and makes him equally thrilled and happy. There is a circuit and exchange which finally perfectly balances and leaves each content.

The man who would be an artist in touch must learn to put this vital elixir into his fingertips, his palms, into the glance of his eyes, suggest it in the tones of his voice, convey it at will from any part of his body which may touch the body of another - yes, even to convey it by mere aura, invisibly, secretly, to another body, near, but not in contact. He must learn to touch with firm and thrilling strength, or with tender gentleness and restfulness. He must learn to stroke and caress with an exquisite delicacy, tactfulness and grace, suggesting music. In the actual embrace he must learn to alternate violent speed and force (yet controlled and never really rude or inconsiderate), in his movements, with touches delicate and soothing, in a contrast of symphonic "storm and peace," which may sink to absolute quietude of strong, tender enfolding.

O touch me, touch me *right!* she said —
(O God, how often womanhood hath said!)
That we two ones as one be wed,
That all with all, throughout, we wed,
Close, close and tender close! she said,
The touch that *knows*, O Man! she said
O touch me, touch me right! she said.

The ideal of the woman should be to apprehend with exquisite intuition every mood of the man almost before he knows it himself and to meet it with sympathy, comprehension and response - relaxing, revivifying, restraining, applauding, reinforcing, encouraging, quieting or thrilling as his need may be. She must realize that her love and admiration are really the psychic basis of the whole relation. The ideal of the man must be to manifest a glorious strength, and passion, held, as a rider would hold a mettled stallion, under an equally glorious control - to prove himself as skillful and chivalrous as heroic. Thus each will be irradiated by the glowing admiration of the other, which is the highest bliss of love.

Probably the most untellably delightful of all human sensations is to touch the flesh of a perfectly mated lover, where the soul is innocent, the heart satisfied, and the magnetic currents seem divinely strong.

There is so much, so *much*,
In human touch!

Cleanness

Always in the sexual life there should be cleanness - that innocence, kindness, justice of feeling which instinctively prefers any sacrifice of immediate passional pleasure rather than befoul or degrade a high ideal, or to jeopardize the physical or spiritual health of the beloved, or of self, or of the tenderly considered, possible unborn.

Cleanness expresses itself in a reverent regard and considerate self-control at all times, concerning all things, thoughts, motions and relations of sex, and the conscientious use of all organs and functions in the service of the soul's ideal.

The clean may be mistaken, but whatever they do they cannot be impure.

Sex and Soul

Sex is very close to soul. Whoso touches sex touches the secrets and centers of life. This is the Mid-Spot, the Origin, the Crux, the Mystery. In sex the soul is naked. At the contacts of sex the soul trembles, quivers, is shaken to its midmost. The voice of sex, in its power, is as the voice of God - the most imperious and certain-to-be-obeyed call known in Nature or to man.

Sex, soul, religion, morality, are not to be separated. They belong together. The first reverence we detect in Nature is that of the male for the female, of offspring for mother. There is fear elsewhere, but here are mysterious adumbrations and blendings of attraction, adoration, worshipful obedience and withdrawing respect. Sex-religion was the first religion of man and we shall never get back again to true religion until we again see God in His creative motions and worship and reverence the soul in flesh.

Sincerity, seriousness, cleanness, generosity and liberty in sex are the foundations of morality. Where these are found we have genuine love, true relations, open souls, fearless hearts, fragrant bodies, healthy children, happy mothers, a society everywhere honest, free and kind. Where these or any of them are lacking, society rots, lies fester, men exist by crime, and shame broods like a cloud.

The agitation of the youth who blushes, trembles and stammers before the woman he loves; of the girl who melts in his arms, not daring to lift her eyes, dumb, soul-shaken, overcome by the mystery of her being and emotions - these reveal by signs ineffable the sacred seriousness of sex.

When Sex Satisfies

For all finer natures, sex relations are only satisfying when touched by moral and religious emotion - when they are serious - when they involve the depths - when they inspire to the heights.

When sex *feels sacred in the use* it gives a divine innocence to the moment, a satisfying sweetness of recollection in the memory.

Sex is only satisfying where it is absolutely free, in a liberty made new and genuine by glad, mutual consent at every moment of its being.

Sex only satisfies when on both sides there are kindness, innocence, consideration - a love that is *goodness in expression*, that *gives* and *blesses*.

Sex only satisfies the finer natures when it unites souls, not merely copulates bodies for a thrill.

An atmosphere of frivolity, recklessness, mere hedonism and indulgence about sex, invariably reacts in disgust — the conscience instantly stamps this as "sin."

Sex having two offices - to unite souls and propagate bodies - there are for these offices two unions - Karezza-union for the deeper love, orgasmal-union for physical begetting. Do not make the mistake of using the latter for the former.

But sex is also like a food, and sexual contact with vital magnetic exchange at certain not-too-long intervals, varying with different temperaments, conditions and times of life, seems necessary for health and satisfying living and is also a perfectly valid and justifying reason for sexual embraces and caresses, even where there is only innocent need on one side and tender kindness on the other, or where on both sides there is only need and kindness.

There is biological reason to suppose that the function of sex to mysteriously feed and rejuvenate is its oldest and perhaps most essential function, antedating its reproductive function a long, long time.

Starting then from the beginning, the functions of sex may be read as three:

- First: to feed and rejuvenate by contact-pressure (perhaps by a sort of catalysis) and a mysterious generation, interchange and mutual exchange of subtle processes and forces.
- Second: physical reproduction - child-creation.
- Third: soul-union, the mystery of love, affection, spiritual-companionship, mental-inspiration.

In all its normal aspects sex is creative and uniting, kind and life-giving in function.

Duality and Spirituality in Sex

Unless we recognize that sex is spiritual as well as physical, we shall not understand how it is the great agent of love. For love is the uniting principle in the universe, and as all things have their opposites, that which reconciles and at-ones them, marries them, is that which we term sex. In the physical organs of male and female, sex is objectified in fixed forms, but this in only one example, and a very small one, of sex. These organs relate peculiarly to physical union and reproduction, but when we come to consider all the various ways in which sex unites and reproduces we find no limitations to these tools. On the contrary, the "duality" which philosophers constantly recognize in Nature is nothing but the larger sex-relation and interaction. All chemical attractions and repulsions, all electrical, are sexual. But we shall not understand this at all if we think always of men and women as such, or of physical males and females when we say sex.

Physical sex-forms are often very deceptive. Some women are more masculine than the average man, and *vice versa*, which accounts for much of the phenomena of homosexuality. In all deep-seated friendships between those of the same external sex it will be observed that spiritually one represents the masculine element, one the feminine. And masculine women normally love and marry feminine men. And when such come together, while his physical sex is male and hers female, so that physically he may impregnate her, she is spiritually male and may spiritually impregnate him and beget spiritual children in his brain and soul (that is, thoughts, ideals, purposes, emotions) that change and rule his whole character.

But the complexity by no means stops here. Each person is dual in sex, both in body and in each organ and part. We still remember our divine ancestry, still are androgyne and hermaphrodite. And this is not only so, but it is variably, changeably so. Sex alternates and plays through us all the time, partly involuntarily, partly as we will it. It varies even with difference in weather, food, fatigue, health, and all external impressions and internal evolutions. Thus one listening to an argument may be altogether negative, receptive, feminine in mind, till some word or thought changes the mood, and then, instantly, positive, projective, masculine - this change of mental sex possible, in the same person of either physical sex, within a few moments of time.

This has a very practical relation to Karezza. In its long, blending, intimate embrace of body and soul a great deal more than the more obvious sex-organs and functions are concerned. A similar sexual interchange takes place between all corresponding parts of body and mind, every function and every thought. Thus while her pelvis may be feminine to his, her bosom may be masculine to his breast; his hands may be more masculine than hers, but her mouth and tongue more positive than his. His intellect may be dominatingly masculine to her mind and yet in emotion and feeling she may control. And this may at any moment be all reversed. And this may be true not only of regions, but of small parts of regions, single muscles or nerves in one being masculine or feminine, according to health or stimulus, without regard to the possibly opposite condition of the surrounding parts. So of every thought, emotion or word. Could anyone view the two lovers physically, I fancy he would see streams of sex-force flowing from each to the other from every part, eagerly received, drunk up and returned, till it would be hard to tell which one was the most masculine or feminine. If the streams of magnetism were objectified to the eye, they would appear like filaments, making the two forms appear to be literally sewn and tied, netted and interwoven together by innumerable millions of little threads of electrical love and commerce. No wonder love is called "attachment."

But more than this - an unconscious change of mood or thought, or a conscious effort of the will, can reverse the sex of any part and make that instantly feminine which before was masculine, or turn feminine to masculine. This may be done skillfully and with delightful effect by those trained in sex-expression. The sexual motions and magnetisms, the touch of the skin, of the hands, the glance of the eyes, the kiss of the lips, the tones of the voice, all these can be instantly reversed from a tender, yielding, clinging, drawing, appealing receptiveness to a bold, positive, thrilling bestowal of vital force. It is plain, then, that the more points on which two lovers are unlike, yet capable of easy and loving exchange, the greater their capacity to give each other joy.

Those who aspire to sexual genius and mastership should take deep note of this, for it is very important: *One's power to give sexual joy and satisfaction depends upon one's power to give one's partner a cup for every stream and a drink for every thirst* - in other words, to give sex-force where the partner's desire is to receive, and to receive sex-force where the partner desires to give. All this can be learned and acquired, just as other controls and other self-directions can be acquired. It is simply tact and adaptation in the realm of sex. The woman who can be sweet, yielding, tender, receptive to the man when he is sexually virile and strong, and motherly, helpful, executive, when he is dispirited and weak, has vastly more sexual charm than one who can only be timid and passive, or who is always assertive and manlike. And the more easily and skillfully these changes can be made in the same embrace, to meet differing moods, exercise different desires, and to prevent monotony, the longer the embrace can continue, the greater its benefits and joy. Karezza is exactly like music - it may be only a rude monotonous rhythm, or mere chant or refrain, or it can attain any perfection of harmonic or symphonic complexity and execution. The character and individuality of the players, their natural genius or "ear" for the changes, and their acquired experience and skill being the determining factors, together with the quality and "tune" of the instruments themselves. Genius in sexual expression is just as normal and certain of occurrence as any other, and some day artists in love will be known and recognized as such — nay, even today, under all our incubus of repression and Grundyism, they are known and admired.

And it will be recognized that the sexual organism, strung with its vibrating and, delicate nerves, is an instrument more perfect than any violin or harp, capable of as exquisite harmonies under the touch of a master. Yet, even as the perfect music is not that which the mere perfection of technique produces, but that into which the true artist breathes his passion and his life, so it is with sex. It is not simply the man of training, the one who knows how, but the man who loves his instrument, and throws the passion and enthusiasm of his soul into the expression, who elicits the divine melody.

All art demands the lover, and sex-art is the art of the lover.

Sex-Commerce and the Elixir of Life

I believe that sex runs through all life, animal and vegetable - perhaps through the inorganic world also. And that the sexes are cannibals, feeding on each other - the sexes are *food* to each other.

I believe that both sexes are in the simplest uni-cell. That, afterwards, as life evolves, there is a tendency to a division of labor - to separate the sexes into two persons, but that always the two sexes are more or less in one - always the male is part female, the female part male in varying degrees of more or less.

I believe that the processes of life require as an essential a frequent, if not constant, interchange of maleness with femaleness. I believe this takes place within the organism constantly and in proportion to its perfection there is beauty and health. In every cell there is this interchange, and between different cells of the organism there is such an exchange.

But just as in-and-in breeding finally "runs out" the strain, and leads to deterioration, so in-and-in exchange of maleness and femaleness - really the same thing - leads to deterioration at last, though many things may assist to delay and postpone the process - change in nourishment, in environment, etc.

Therefore the maleness of one person needs exchange with the femaleness of some other person; the femaleness of one with the maleness of another.

Homosexuality bases partly on the fact that this exchange may be effected, with more or less satisfaction, sometimes, with persons of the same sex (who, as both sexes are in one, are more or less persons of the opposite sex also) but this too is a form of in-and-in exchange, therefore the normal and best exchange is with persons whose sex is visibly and predominantly opposite to one's own. Man normally goes to woman, woman to man. And even here very opposite temperaments are usually preferred, the smooth by the hairy, the red-headed by the black-haired, the fat, by the lean, etc., because these have existed under very different environments, have fed on different nourishment, which they exchange through sex, and, so still further put away in-and-in exchange and complement each other's lacks - Nature always seeking an equilibrium and redistribution of elements in alternation.

This exchange and mutual feeding can be effected in any way in which the sexes can come into each other's aura, but it is most easily effected by touch, and most perfectly by the complete union of Karezza. The sexual orgasm having an entirely different purpose, that is, not the nourishment of the two individuals concerned, but the transmission of life and nourishment to another, a new and third organism starting from these two, tends rather to defeat and prevent the nourishment of the two, and is normally limited, usually, to propagation. To indulge in the orgasm frequently, as a mere pleasure and indulgence, is to create a vice - salacity.

I do not pretend to know what this sexual food is. We may theorise that it is a "flux of electrons," a "current of corpuscles," "hormones," or what not - who knows? - but its effects we may see. The thrill, the vigor, the brilliancy, the glow of lovers; the "illusion," the "glamour," the "romance" of love we all know. This means swift exchange and joyous feasting. Suppose we call this food the Elixir of Life?

But the mere suggestion of this sexual exchange seems to marvelously quicken and benefit even the inward in-and-in exchanges. Thus reading a love letter, or a love story, handling a keepsake, thinking of a lover, and a thousand other such things, may benefit the whole being by sex suggestion.

There are those who claim that the cells of the animal organism go to seed and that each one of these little molecules, or corpuscles, go to the ova or spermatozoa to represent that cell in the new organism to be formed by reproduction, so that the essence of everything in the parent organism may be in the offspring. And there are Karezza-ites who explain the thrill and exhilaration of Karezza by claiming that during its exercise these vital seed-elements, not being thrown off by an orgasm, are thrown, instead, into the circulation again and become a nerve food and cell-elixir; perhaps leading to the return to the germ or sperm of new seed-elements more vivified and electric than before. And that this explains why the mere autosuggestion of love, above alluded to, if intense enough, by somewhat the same process, seems to vitalize like Karezza.

This may not ultimately prove scientific, but I am inclined to accept it and reconcile it with the preceding - to believe that love is a process of self-feeding and redistribution of elements within the organism as well as of mutual feeding and exchange between lovers.

And I believe that all human love that naturally seeks expression in embracing is, at least largely, moved by and based upon this human need of vital exchange and sexual rejuvenation.

Moreover, morally, we need to recognize that this desire of the sexes for hugging, kissing, caressing, contact, closeness and the most pressing and intimate touch, is not vicious or suspicious, but a physiological, a *food* desire. One needs meats of sexual touch, just as one needs meals of food, only not so often. The fullest life cannot be lived without them. However, there can be sexual gluttony, just as there can be food gluttony. And there can be foul, poisonous, unhealthy sexual touches and contacts, just as there can be poisonous, foul, unhealthy viands. Intelligence, selection, self-control, refinement, hygienic wisdom and education, and a sensitive conscience, are needed with both. But neither should be regarded from the attitude of prejudice or mere sentiment, or convention, but from that of science, common sense and the ideal.

The Wine of Sex

The sexual elixir, essence, magnetism, whatever it is, in the human blood, is the true natural stimulant and joy-giver of life. It is this that gives the "illusion," the "glamour," the romance," the "blindness," the "madness," the "thrill," and all the rest of which the lore of love tells us. All other stimulants are artificial - this one is absolutely natural; all other stimulants are poisons - this one is food; all others have reactions, are finally narcotics and depressants - this one has no reactions; reaction only appears in its absence, when it is lost or wasted.

It is courage, wit, sparkle, radiance, imagination, high spirits, enthusiasm, creative-passion, religious fervor - everything that lifts life above the clod and the monotonous levels. It is the inspiration, directly or indirectly, of almost every poem, song, painting, or other work of art. It has led more men to battle than any bugle note or national peril. It is the great kindler and sustainer of ideals.

Very few understand this or realize it sufficiently. It is commonly observed how lovers glow and radiate and move in an enchanted world; but this is all attributed to love itself. On the contrary, it is the wine of sex that gives love its enchantment and divine dreams. This is easily proven by giving lovers unrestricted license to express their transports. No sooner have they wasted the wine of sex by reckless embraces - often a single orgasm will thus temporarily demagnetize the man - though they love each other just the same, as they will each stoutly assert - the irresistible attraction and radiance and magnetic thrills are gone, and there is a strange drop into cool, critical intellection or indifference, or perhaps dislike. But as the wine of sex reaccumulates and lifts again in the glass, the old magic and charm reappear.

And in this is a clear natural lesson as to the inestimable value of this elixir in human life and in the ethics of the love-life itself. The one thing that makes life worth living is not its cold facts, but the romantic glow and glamour with which a vivid and kindled imagination invests them, and any manner of conducting the love-life which can create and maintain this zest and charm at its highest is clearly the ethical one. Ascetics, perceiving only that the sex forces give inspiration and that orgasms waste them, and wrongly arguing that in sex life sexual waste is inevitable, teach that the sexes should avoid each other and turn all sex forces into channels of ambition, public service, religion, etc. This is like telling a man that he should give all his money for the public good, but should avoid earning any; fails to recognize that it takes sexual consciousness, sexual association to develop sexual force. Others, going a step further, getting a glimmer of this last, urge that the sexes associate, but Platonically only. These fail to see that to hold a delicious cup constantly to the lips of a thirsty man and yet forbid him to drink, is to waste his force in needless cravings and foolish battles to subdue them and finally usually ends in failure and a sickening sense of guilt.

On the other hand, to have frequent orgasmal embraces, as most married lovers do, is to keep the wine in the sexual lovers low by constant spilling, to thus kill all romance and delight and finally starve and tire out love itself.

Here comes in the application and immense value of Karezza. It is perfect self-control, and yet, once understood and rightly practiced, it is such a perfect and complete satisfaction to all the nerves and appetites concerned that all sense of denial or restriction is lost in one of higher, larger, sweeter expression. It brews and fills every vessel with the sexual wine of ambition, charm, enchantment, as nothing else can, and maintains it steadily at a high tide, preventing all losses by preventing all reaction, thus making life continuous romance, genius and joy.

It avoids alike the waste of starvation and the waste of excess, the wastefulness of self-torture and self-battle to overcome a perfectly natural and wholesome hunger for sexual contact and closeness - it not only avoids all these wastes, it cultivates the grape and presses the wine into the cup of life which is alone capable of giving man normal inspiration and poetic happiness.

The Karezza Method

Whoso would succeed with Karezza must begin with the mental and spiritual values. Both the man and the woman, and perhaps especially the woman, must resolve that they do not *wish* the orgasm - that there is a greater spiritual and physical unity and emotional bliss to be obtained without it, besides the sense of safety. This must be the fixed thought and ideal of Karezza.

If you are novices, choose a time when you can both be all alone, unhurried and free from interruptions. Concentrate yourselves entirely on your love and joy and the blending of yourselves into one.

Let the room be warm, the surroundings pleasant and esthetic; and be as unhampered by clothing as possible. Let both of you think more about your love than your passion; translate your sex-passion as much as possible into heart-passion; be sensitively alive to the charm of each other's forms, tones, touch and fragrances; let the thought of mutual tenderness and blessing never leave you for an instant, and make everything that you do and say and feel and think religious in its purity, idealism, aspiration. If you do not come nearer heaven in this act and relation, than in anything else you do or ever will do, you fail of perfect Karezza.

Let your embrace be music and a living poem.

Now to you, the man, I speak: Lie down beside your partner and begin to caress her gently with the softness of your hands and fingertips. Tell her to relax herself and lie utterly passive. Tell her to yield herself to the bliss of utter peace and realization. Tell her that you love her and that your whole being longs for entire unity with her. Remember that you cannot use the word "love" too often. She will never tire of it and it is your watchword. Be to her an incarnate blessing. Try to convey God to her.

As your hands caress her, tell her how beautiful her features are to you - her brow, her hair, her lips, her throat - her arms, hands, bosom, waist, the flowing rounded lines of her limbs. Grow eloquent, poetic in her praise. The Loved One can never be too much praised or appreciated by the Lover. Spend plenty of time on these preparatory caresses.

Finally your touch will grow near and you will come to the focus of all, "the love-flesh" - the Flower. Be tender; be tender, for this is Holiness itself - the seal of God on the woman's person.

If there is dew and moisture here, a flowing with honey, you may begin - that is if your own Finger of Love is firm and fit.

Let there be no hurry or thought of rudeness - be tender, be tender! Have her lie in a straight line, easy, at peace, utterly relaxed and willing.

Begin, seeing to it that the lips do not enfold to prevent. Be gentle, tender, steady, steady. Keep your thoughts on love, not passion. Let her help you by doing the same and murmuring to you, "I love you!" If your passion threatens to overcome you, pause and sublimate it into tenderness of love. Feel strong and confident and say, "I can!" Maintain your own positiveness. Feel yourself stronger than she is, than your passions are. But above all think of your spiritual love. Let her be utterly relaxed physically, let her hold the thought of Peace. Yet for her to hold the thought "I will help him!" *would help.* Do not worry and do not mind how long you have to wait before strength and self-control return and you can go on. Finally the stress subsides and you can continue. If she suffers pain, caress her with your hands, pity her, and be tender and very sympathetic, but reassure her and go on. She herself does not wish you to stop or to fail. Reassure and help each other. When you do finally pass the gates and enter the Hall of the Feast and the Holy of Holies, the worst of the battle will be over and self-control much easier. Penetration can now be perfect and complete.

Now let her put her arms around you and sweetly kiss you, but with heart-love, not yet passion. Pour out your soul to her in extravagance of out-gushing, poetic love. Praise her with every epithet you can honestly use. Give her your soul's best, always your best - and call out the best and purest from her.

At other times - and this is most important - be silent and quiet, but try to feel yourself a magnetic battery, with the Finger of Love as the positive pole, and pour out your vital electricity to her and consciously direct it to her womb, her ovaries, her breasts, lips, limbs, everywhere filling her in every nerve and fiber with your magnetism, your life, love, strength, calmness and peace. This attitude of *magnetation* is the important thing in Karezza, its secret of sweetest success. In proportion as you acquire the habit and power of withdrawing the electric qualities from your sexual stores and giving them out in blessing to your partner from your sex-organs, hands, lips, skin, everywhere; from your eyes and the tones of your voice; will you acquire the power to diffuse and bestow the sex-glory, envelop yourselves in its halo and aura, and to satisfy yourself and satisfy her without an orgasm. Soon you will not even think of self-control, because you will have no desire for the orgasm, nor will she. You will both regard it as an awkward and interrupting accident. And the practice of Magnetation will beautify and strengthen every organ in your body that you thus use to express it, as well as hers. It is the great beautifier. Every look from your eyes, yes, every touch of your hands, and the tones of your voice will become vibrant with magnetic charm.

And while you are magnetizing her, try to feel your utter unity with her. This is the real ideal and end of Karezza. You will finally enter into such unity that in your fullest embrace you can hardly tell yourselves apart and can read each other's thoughts. You will feel a physical unity as if her blood flowed in your veins, her flesh were yours. For this is the Soul-Blending Embrace.

If any part of her is weak or ill you can direct the magnetic currents there with the conscious thought of healing.

But this is anticipation and a description of the perfect thing. Perhaps at first you will have much difficulty and many failures. If while you are penetrating you feel the orgasm irresistibly approaching, withdraw entirely, lift yourself a little higher up and have the emission against her body, while you are pressed close to her warmth and consoling love. After all is over, wipe all away, carefully, with a convenient cloth, and be very careful that no drops can reach her entrance. Then repose quietly by her side, talking tenderly and lovingly. Do not worry — all will come right - this is only a common accident with beginners and to be expected - perhaps with the very passionate and fully-sexed, several times in succession. Remember you are not yet used to each other or in magnetic rapport. If she is a true woman she will never reproach you, but will be all patience, sympathy, loyally working with you to attain the perfect result.

At the end of an hour, not sooner, all discharges having long since passed and dried up, if you can again feel potent it will be safe to renew the attempt. [1] Caress her for a while, exactly as at first, and be sure her nectar-moisture and willingness are as at first. This is your sign of invitation - of her blissful welcome and Nature's chrism. If she is dry, you will hurt her. The top having been taken off your passion by the emission, you will probably, this time, feel less pressure and be able to easily succeed, but the second testicle may demand equal privileges and again you may fail. Do exactly as at first and so continue till you do succeed. Practice makes perfect and "it's dogged that does it," Thackeray said. Never permit yourself to contemplate anything but ultimate and ideal success. It is right here, after one or two failures, that most men give up and declare the whole thing impossible. Yet it is right here, and after such failures, that success becomes easiest, because the discharges have lessened the seminal pressure. If the attempt is renewed just as often as potency can be renewed, success is certain. Any man can succeed if he will persevere.

When you have fully acquired the power you will go on from strength to strength. You will amaze yourself and your partner by what is easily possible to you. You will be able to make any motion you please, that anybody can make anywhere, yet with no failures. You can take the most unusual positions and change places with your partner. You can allow her to be as active as she pleases, or to have the orgasm herself, if she greatly desires it, with no danger to your equilibrium. You can continue the embrace for half an hour, an hour, or even two hours. You can repeat it twice, or perhaps three times, in twenty-four hours, with no sensation of excess. And, so on. But keep the spiritual on top, dominant - loving is the first thing, and at-one-ment in the highest fruition of your souls, your real end. Sex-passion as an end in itself will degrade you. Make it a tool of your spirit.

Karezza is *the* embrace - The Embrace - the most perfect and satisfying thing in human life, between two mates who truly love. All other caresses point to this and are unsatisfactory because they are not it. It is the only embrace for the truly refined and poetic, as an adequate expression of their insatiable longing to be at one. It is Heaven, on earth.

[1] To facilitate this — immediately after the emission stroke, with a firm, gentle pressure, upward from the anus to the scrotum, thus aiding complete discharge, and thereafter soon urinate.

The Woman's Part in Karezza

The opinion prevails that in Karezza the man does it all and the woman's co-operation is negligible. This error may have arisen in part from the old name, "Male Continence," for the method.

On the contrary, her co-operation, or at least acquiescence, is indispensable, and it is probable that a reckless woman, or one who deliberately and skillfully seeks to do so, can break the control of the most expert man in the art.

For instance, very sudden and unexpected leaps, plunges, or contortions on the woman's part, or wild and abandoned writhings are difficult to withstand, and there is one particular movement, in which the feminine organs clasp tenaciously their sensitive guest and then are drawn suddenly, powerfully backward and downward, which, if executed quickly and voluptuously enough and repeated, I feel sure must unlock the strongest man living.

Also where the woman's muscles are tense and she is quivering and vibrating within with avid hunger almost past control, radiating a thrilling excitement - to attempt entrance at such a moment almost certainly means an explosion, though the same condition after penetration is perfect and a harmonious rapport established, may be supportable, safe and exquisitely delightful, provided the man's own will or passion is still stronger.

Karezza should always begin gently. Too intense or excited a condition on either side, but especially on the woman's side, at the very outset, militates against success. As a rule the woman, at first, should be in a state of complete muscular relaxation. Strong passion *in her feeling* is not only permissible but excellent, if it is under complete control, if the muscles are not tensed by it, and if it is wisely and helpfully wielded. There is a passion which grips and dominates its subject, greedy, jerky, avid and, as it were, hysterical - like the food-appetite which bolts its meal. This makes Karezza impossible. But there is another passion just as strong, or stronger, more consciously delightful, in which the emotion is luxurious, voluptuous, esthetic, epicurean, which lingers, dallies, prolongs and appreciates, which is neither hurried nor excited, and which invites all the joys and virtues to the feast. This is the passion of true Karezza, especially of the woman who is perfect in the art. She is then to her lover like music, like a poem, not like a bacchante or a neurotic.

As a rule the woman's passion, however great, must be subordinated to the man's. He must feel himself the stronger and more positive of the two and as controlling the situation. If the woman takes the lead, is more positive, especially if she assumes this suddenly and unexpectedly, the result is almost always failure. The woman may rule in the house, in the business, in the social life, and it may be very well, but in Karezza the man must be her chief and her hero or the relation leaves both dissatisfied. In the ordinary, orgasmal, procreative embrace the woman may dominate and be successful, at least become impregnated, though her pleasure is usually imperfect, but Karezza is a different matter. And this is because in Karezza the woman is happy in proportion to her fulfilled femininity, the man in proportion to his realized masculinity, and each happy in realizing this in the intimate touch of the other.

There is a physical help which the woman may render at the very outset which is important. It often happens at the beginning of penetration that the labia, one or both of them, are infolded, or pushed in, acting as an impediment and lessening pleasure or causing a disagreeable sensation. If the woman, before penetration begins, will, with her fingers, reach in and open wide the lips, drawing them upward and outward the fullest extent, she will greatly facilitate entrance, and if she will several times repeat this during the Karezza, each time drawing the inner labia outward, while her partner presses inward, it will be found greatly to increase the contact surface and conscious enjoyment, giving a greater sense of ease and attainment.

If a woman by intuitional genius or acquired skill does the right thing, her passion is a food and a stimulus to the man, filling him with a triumphant pride. He is lifted, as it were, by a deep tide, on which he floats buoyantly and exultantly, like a seabird on a wave. Under such conditions both parties become exalted by an enthusiasm approaching ecstasy, a feeling of glorious power and perfect safety no words can adequately describe. And this, I insist, depends mainly on the woman.

Under such conditions of realized power and ability almost any movements, on either side, are possible, provided they are ordinary, expected, and carrying a sort of rhythm. Remember that Karezza is, in its way, a form of the dance. But no movement should be too often repeated without a break. Change is in every way pleasing and desirable. Steady repetition excites to the orgasm, or tires, satiates, chafes or bruises. No movement at any time should be jerky or unexpectedly sudden. Lawless, nervous, unregulated flouncings and wrigglings should be barred as from a waltz. They properly belong to epileptic states of the orgasmal embrace, and for that very reason have no place in Karezza, which is the opposite. There should be often, long, tender, restful pauses - alternations of "storm and peace," as one woman happily phrased it - and in many cases the whole embrace may most helpfully be very quiet. This part should be decided by the woman and as she wishes it.

The mental attitude and atmosphere and the words of the woman are of inestimable importance. As before said, she must hold the thought that she does not wish or will the orgasm and that she will help the man to avoid it. She should feel calm, strong, confident, safe and pure. At such a time a sensitive man will almost know her thoughts and participate in her emotions, and her sub-consciousness, and his, affect each other like mingling streams. Nervousness, doubt, remorse, suspicion, irritation, guilt, coldness, repulsion or blame may make him impotent for the time. Too tense or avid a passion may do the same, or pull the trigger of discharge. Her attitude should always, consistently, be one of encouragement. The sudden, perhaps sub-conscious fear that the woman is expecting more than he can give, and will blame him if he fail, often quite destroys a sensitive man's courage and makes temporary impotence or an emission inevitable, where admiration and approval could develop a sexual hero. Nothing else can possibly help a man so much as to feel all around him the glow of his loved one's loving admiration and trust, her comfort, satisfaction and confidence. Her praise is iron and wine to him.

She need not say much, but if there are few words they must be eloquent. Some women make little, inarticulate musical sounds of applause and joy. Any way she must make him understand, and the chief thing to understand is that the love-side is of a thousand times more importance to her than the sex-side - and this especially if, for the time, he has failed.

There is probably no place in the love-life where an attitude and effort of generous love - a soul-cry of "I will help him! I will praise him! I will love him!" will return so much in personal profit and pleasure to the woman as right here.

The woman must feel innocent - that she is doing right. To accept an embrace under conditions of moral self-reproach may sicken a sensitive partner as well as herself, and cause him genital injury.

Remember that Karezza is passionate emotion guided by the intellect and sweetened by the sanction of the soul. It is an art and belongs to the world of the beautiful. It is because it is so controlled and sanctioned that it appeals so to the higher minds - the noble, the poetic and the refined. Exactly as music and poetry exploit some emotional episode in beautiful detail of rhythmic expression long drawn out, so Karezza exploits, in the rhythmic, changeful figures of a clinging dance, the beauty and bliss of the sexual episode.

Karezza is the art of love in its perfect flower, its fulfillment of the ideal dream.

The Woman's Time of Great Desire

The desire of a woman is seldom so comparatively constant and steady as with a man, but fickle and variable, often latent, though the practice in Karezza tends to equalize the sexes in this, but there are times when, from various reasons, a wave of intense craving suddenly sweeps over her. Particularly is this likely to happen just before the appearance of the menses. And at such times the woman's desire is very likely to exceed in wild, fiery force that of an ordinary man. Wherefore it follows that very few women at such times get complete satisfaction, leading to great disappointments and marital unhappiness. The unexpected violence of the woman's emotion, upsets the man's nerves and causes either a "too quick" orgasm, or complete psychic impotence.

Now I think the Karezza-man seldom has any difficulty with the woman whose desire he has himself aroused by caresses and wooing. But when the desire arises spontaneously in her, her natural tendency appears to be to abandon herself to it, to abdicate all self-control, forget everything else and recklessly, fiercely, almost madly demand sensual gratification. This attitude is a very difficult one indeed for the Karezza-lover to meet, because just in proportion to his fineness, sensitiveness and real fitness to be a Karezza artist is his susceptibility, almost to telepathy, to the woman's moods. If he meets her on her own plane, the orgasm cannot be refused, while if he struggles against her for his Karezza ideal, he is almost certain in the conflict either to lose his poise or to become impotent. This is because this wild desire on her part is normally related to reproduction and is intended by Nature to overcome any male scruples and lead to an immediate embrace and swift orgasm, followed by conception. If, however, the woman wills to have it met on the Karezza plane, and converted into an esthetic love-embrace, then she herself must take the initiative and put it on that plane. She must begin the process by getting an inclusive grip on herself, relaxing her tense muscles and steadying her quivering nerves. And no longer concentrating altogether on the sexual, she must sublimate a portion of her passion into heart-love, into a tender desire to encourage her lover and assist him to complete success. The man, whose nerves have been thrown into agitation by her un-governed attitude and thrilling vibrations, will recover courage and assurance the moment he senses the aid of her self-control, and his proud power will return when her eyes turn admiringly upon him and her tone and her touch give him her confidence and the cooperating sup-port of her strength.

The wise woman, skillful and trained in her art, will thus beautifully control herself until the man has attained complete and deepest union with her, and the blending current of their mutual magnetism is smoothly running, and then will gradually, as he can bear it, turn on her bat-teries full strength, reinforcing and redoubling his, till all need of restraint disappears and she may let herself go to her uttermost of bliss and expression, to the limit of com-plete satiety.

No other time affords an embrace so completely satisfy-ing to the woman as this, so full of joy to both, capable of reaching such heights of ecstasy, but to realize this she must understand that it is up to her to furnish her full half or more in skillful assistance and magnetic contribution. A woman should be ashamed to expect the man alone to be the Karezza-artist. She should take pride in her own superb sex-power, the poetry of her rhythms, the artistry of her acts. She should have an exulting delight in proving herself worthy of his adoration as the Queen of Love.

And always this should be remembered: The more heart-love the more sex-joy.

Does the Woman Need the Orgasm?

A lady physician of my acquaintance thinks that a woman would be left congested in her sexual organs, probably, by Karezza, did she not have the orgasm, and the result would finally be disease.

I have not found it so in practice, and the criticism would almost appear to have come from one who had not known Karezza in its perfect form. If valid, it would apply to the man as well and would destroy all force of the case for Karezza for either sex, which is far from what my critic desires.

In Dr. Max Huner's *Disorders of the Sexual System*, a work in which the woman's need of the orgasm is strongly insisted on, I find these significant words: "'Whenever a woman states that she remains dry after coitus it generally means a lack of orgasm." In other words, it is very common in the ordinary orgasmal embrace, for the man to have an orgasm in a few moments and depart, leaving the woman entirely unsatisfied in every way. The ordinary husband-and-wife embrace, anyway, is purely sexual, and based on his demand to get rid of a surplus. There is little or no thought to make it esthetic or affectional - it is merely animal. If the husband stays long enough and excites his wife sufficiently to have an orgasm, then she has a gushing out of fluids that relieves the congestion brought on by his approaches, and on the physical plane, at least, she is relieved and satisfied, the same as he. If not, "she remains dry." Her moisture or dryness, then, are a pretty good index of her physical satisfaction and relief of congestion, or the reverse.

But what happens in Karezza? Here, if she really loves her partner, her whole nature is attuned to his, in delicious docility, expectation and rapport. Every nerve vibrates in sweet gratitude and response to his touch. There is a marvelously sweet blending and reconciliation of the voluptuous and the spiritual that satisfies both her body and her soul at once and makes her exquisitely sensitive to everything poetic or esthetic in his acts. In this state, when interrelation has been successfully established and his magnetism is flowing through her every fiber, uniting them as one, such a heavenly ecstasy of peace, love and happiness possesses her that she "melts" (there is no other word for it), her whole being wishes to join with his, and though there is no orgasm in the ordinary definition of the word yet her fluids gush out in an exactly similar manner and all possible congestion is utterly and completely relieved. Not only is this true of the mucus membranes, but the outer skin also is bathed in a sweet sweat. Indeed I consider mutual perspiration as very desirable, if not almost indispensable to the most perfect magnetation, as the moist bodies in loving contact seem to communicate the magnetic, electric currents so much more effectually then.

Rest assured that no woman who has known Karezza in its ideal, its "Heaven" and "Peace" form, remains dry, nor is she left with any trace of congestion, or restlessness. On the contrary, she often sinks into a blissful slumber in the very midst of the embrace, just after its sweetest delights.

In truth I have often thought that a very plausible argument might be advanced for the claim that in Karezza the woman really did have an orgasm, only in such a very gradual form, spread over so long a time, and so sweetly sublimated and exalted in love, that the usual symptoms did not appear or were unrecognized as such.

Psychic Impotence

This book would be incomplete were I to make no mention of that sudden and mysterious loss of erectile power which sometimes befalls men. Perhaps there are few men who do not know the secret dread of some day becoming impotent.

I remember a champion athlete - a magnificent man physically - confessing to me that he was afraid to marry, fearing that he would not be able to satisfy his wife. And perhaps the earliest sexual story that I remember was that of a soldier, in the time of the Civil War, who by a sudden and natural motion lost his power, which no effort of himself or his mistress could restore. All my life such tales have come to me. Tragic tales, some of them, as where a spiteful woman overwhelmed her helpless lover with shame and reproach; where divorce was demanded for this cause; where a marriage between two devoted lovers remained unconsummated to the end, the husband dying in a few years, perhaps of a broken heart. These and many others. Who has not heard of the pitiful case of Carlyle and his Jane Welsh, as told by Froude? And it has been hinted that the same cause lay back of Ruskin's beautiful surrender of his wife to the artist Millais, and of the relation of Swift to his Stella and Vanessa.

The mystery of this thing lies in its suddenness and un-accountability. No wonder that in the superstitious it has suggested witchcraft. If it came only to cowards, to weaklings, to the sterile, to bashful boys and inexperienced lovers, it would not be so strange. But precisely these may never be troubled by it, while a Don Juan of experience and proud list of conquests; a hero of courage; or a Titan of genius, whose virile mind dominates his time, may suddenly be stricken by it, perhaps blasted for life. It may occur with one woman and not with another, at one time and not another, or it may appear permanent and incurable.

The very worst of it is the mental effect upon the victim. For ages the man human has dreaded to be called "impotent." His manly power is the dearest attribute of man. There are no words to describe the agony, the shame, the bitter self-reproach, the helplessness, the awful despair; that may overwhelm an innocent, loving and otherwise perfect man when the fear comes upon him that his virility has left him and that he may perhaps always disappoint and appear a weakling in the eyes of the woman whose embraces may be dearer and more desired than aught else in life. Just as nothing else gives a man such pride, courage, inspiration and exaltation as to be able to perfectly embrace and satisfy the woman he loves, so nothing else has such power to crush, sadden, sicken and embitter a man as sexual failure. It drives many and many a man to solitude, old-bachelorhood, misanthropy, misogyny, insanity or suicide. How much of the bitterness and gall of Carlyle's writings may have come from this and the agony of his volcanic and morbid soul under its torture, who can tell?

Now because of the sufferings of my sex from this cause and, incidentally, of the women who love them, I have written this chapter. And it is because I wish to speak a helping word that I preface it with the frank confession (which I would otherwise dread to make) that I have myself, at different times and places, suffered enough from this nervous inability to give me a vivid glimpse of its tortures and a true sympathy with its victims. Even a very few and fleeting experiences can do this. Therefore I have studied it, with a personal as well as general interest. And believe my conclusions are of value.

And first I want to correct many common misconceptions. Psychic impotence, though of course not normal, is not pathologic. It is not a proof of ill health. It is not an evidence of weakness, even of sexual weakness. I speak positively when I say that the man completely impotent at night may be absolutely potent in the morning, or *vice versa*, the man who fails with one woman may within the hour be a marvel of manly power with another. It is not a proof of a lack of love but often of the opposite. It is not in the least an evidence of sterility. A man quite sterile may have no trace of psychic impotence and the man troubled by it may be most virile. I knew a man who completely failed with his wife for some nine or ten months after marriage, who finally became the father of four children and is now a grandfather. It is not a proof of inexperience, for it may occur at any time to any man, after any number of years' experience. Thus Forel says: It is often produced suddenly at the time of marriage in persons who have hitherto been very capable, even in Don Juans." I knew a widower, the father of two children, who married a second time, found himself impotent and never overcame it with that woman. At the time of his death, his wife, though she had been that for years (and their life otherwise was most loving) was still a virgin.

So let no man shame himself for this thing, and let no woman despise her lover for it.

Whatever it is, it depends nearly always upon the action and reaction of the two natures brought together upon each other when in a state of sexual nervousness, or upon some strong mental or subjective impression, checking or diverting the normal nerve stimulus which causes the potent expression of manly power. Thus even with those already in successful embrace, a keenly enjoyed joke, a startling sound from without, an argument, an angry word, or a preoccupying conversation, may suddenly and completely cut off the current.

But usually it seems to arise from autosuggestion, or from some suggestions derived, unconsciously or consciously, from the woman. I say "unconsciously" because I am persuaded that there is much that passes between two lovers of which their brains and conscious egos know nothing. I am inclined to believe that there is a telepathy and clairvoyance between their subjective minds and even between their sexual systems of which their consciousness takes no note. I am satisfied that the sexual nature of the woman may love a man when her mind is convinced that she does not love him - that her sex may desire him while her heart refuses. She may feel an almost irresistible impulse to yield herself to a man whom her soul fears and loathes. Or she may love a man mentally, spiritually, even with a heart-love, to whom her sex is cold and indifferent. Human life is nowadays very complex.

And this is why it is that the most sensitive, refined, intuitive men are the most likely to suffer from psychic impotence. The coarse, sensual, selfish man, concerned only with his own passions and their glut, is little likely to feel it. The man who asks only opportunity, not consent, the man who can rape, is safe from it. But the man who reverences womanhood, the man who adores his mistress, the man deeply and passionately in love, so that every thought and suggestion from his loved one sways him like a compelling power, is easily overcome. We must remember that there is probably no time when a strong man is so utterly suggestible as when he is completely in love. His whole nature is then melted, sensitive, impressible (especially by Her) to a degree otherwise impossible with him.

This is why usually coarse men temporarily exalted by a great love may spend a whole evening in the close companionship of a beloved and reverenced woman and never consciously think of sex. This is why a man hitherto perfectly successful with prostitutes and voluptuous women (who appeal only to sex-passion) when he comes to the bridal-bed with some shrinking and nervous and spiritual girl, who knows nothing of sex and to whom the heart love is everything, may suddenly find his sex efforts imperfect. The very nervousness and fright of his companion, her ignorance, her excitement, her dread of the unknown thing about to happen, all this may react on a man and quite unnerve him, and all the more in proportion to his real love for and rapport with her. Often at such a time the excitement, fatigue and dread of the girl have taken away all sex desire from her and she only fears being hurt, and this sex negativeness may infect her lover subconsciously and demagnetize him. Even where the beginning is all right a single cry of pain from the bride may unman the groom. How can he go on and hurt her!

A woman should know that impotence is often the greatest proof a man can offer of the depth, purity and spirituality of his love for her, of his tenderness and consideration and of the probability of his being a life-long lover.

For we must remember that heart-love, spiritual love, that dear and tender at-one-ing and companioning which romantic love now idealizes and desires, represents an evolution. The original love was simply fierce sexual passion, hungry, physical, selfish, concerned only with its own gratification. And to this day these two loves are generally combined in very various degrees, with the co-ordination between them by no means perfect. It is often difficult to get just the right balance and proportion and requires the wise cooperation of both, something not likely to occur at first - especially in the new, strange conditions of a first conjugation between hitherto sexual strangers, particularly if the woman has for many years known nothing of or repressed the sex-life, and has become moody, abnormal and hypersensitive, or lacks normal sensation, or if the man is very sensitive and deeply in love. There is likely to occur an unbalance and dislocation of the sexual elements with strange results.

Very often it would be better if, for the first night, or for many nights, there was no effort made toward sexual congress, but only toward full expression of the caressive heart-love, until such time as both were consciously ripe and could no longer be denied.

The great danger of an initial failure with a nervous, sensitive and impressible man, is that he may be seized with panic, a terror that the heaven opening to him may be closed forever; that his dear one must be disappointed; that she may despise and cease to love him, perhaps even come to loathe him; or that he must live on under the shame of her pity and unsatisfied longings; that his masculine fellows may come to know of it and ridicule him as no man - and all the other terrors that an excited imagination can conjure up; and that this fear and conviction may be stamped in and fixed by auto-suggestion upon his subconsciousness, making his fear a fact. Sometimes the counter-suggestion of hypnotism, in these cases, becomes the only cure.

One of the most mysterious variants of this trouble is where the woman's desire is unusually, perhaps abnormally strong and passionate, and the man thrilled with an equal desire, finds himself helpless. This is difficult to explain, but I think it will usually be found in these cases that the woman is one who by reason of' her changeable moods, previous cruelty, or something of that sort, has produced a subjective fear in the man. In such temperaments, if not immediately answered and satisfied, the woman will sometimes fly into a nervous rage, covering her disappointing partner with shame and, cruel reproach, or withdrawing her favors in cold contempt. Even if not conscious of this fear it may affect a man, or it may exist as a race-memory, and act on his subconsciousness. In some cases I think the sudden nymphomania of the woman causes disturbed nervous vibrations which upset the nervous balance of the man. But I admit there are some examples of this form, for which I have as yet no explanation. The consoling fact is that this form is usually very ephemeral and occasional only.

Sometimes the heart-love is so strong and motherly in a woman, that the man comes completely under its dominance, and though the two may have great happiness and even sensuous joy in each other's embraces, the local sex-organs fail to become completely aroused. This is particularly likely to happen in a woman no longer young, who is near the turn of life, and is quite normal.

Now as the causes of this thing are mostly psychic, so should the remedies be. Nourishing diet, especially of shellfish, milk, eggs, may assist; running, horseback riding and muscle-beating over the lower spine, nates, [1] hips, thighs, and abdomen, by way of a local tonic; with abundant sleep. But the chief need is to establish the right relation between the psychic natures of the lovers themselves. Especially does this depend upon the woman. If she is patient, tender, loving, considerate; if she can prove to him that she is so happy in his tenderness, his unity, his devotion, that the sex-union is really a very secondary and comparatively unimportant matter with her and she can wait any necessary time for its consummation without distress; especially if she daintily and wisely cultivates in herself a touch of the coquettish, sensuous, voluptuous - appealing subtly and luxuriously to his passions and their stimulus — success is seldom long in coming.

There is nothing that so arouses, supports and sustains the normal sex-passion in a man as for a strongly-sexed woman to fill her aura toward him with a strong, steady, self-controlled appeal - tender, loving, admiring, yet deliciously sensuous and esthetically voluptuous; pure, yet deep, warm, alluring. To most men this is an instant and permanent cure. The lover is lifted as a strong swimmer is by some deep and briny tide, and floats deliciously at ease, bathed in bliss, and in the consciousness of perfect power.

But a nervous, hysterical, moody woman; now frantic, now frigid; often plays strange pranks with the sex-power of a susceptible man.

And the man must, whatever happens, maintain his courage, self-respect and faith in his own manhood, and love and work wisely on till the tide comes in.

More and more as man becomes less dominating, less simply carnal, more sensitive, refined and at one with the woman he loves, will power to initiate, direct and sustain his sex-life and love-expression, to make, mar or mould him emotionally, be hers. And woman should be very glad that this is so. The love-life should be hers. This power is her opportunity, her shield, her glory, and the evidence of the greatness of her soul is in the wisdom of her use of it.

And just as this spot is the most vulnerable in a man's whole life, the place where he can be most deeply and in-curably wounded, even so is the depth and eternal quality of his gratitude to the woman who continues to love him despite his weakness, and assists him back to pride and power.

I remember one beautiful instance of this that came to my knowledge. A handsome and brilliant young man, weakened in this way, attracted the sympathy of a woman who devotedly called out, cultivated and restored his power. And though she was very plain, a woman of many faults, un-popular, and many years his senior, he adhered to her ever afterward with a faithfulness and gratitude that nothing could mar. He no doubt felt that she had done more than save his life - she had made it worthwhile to live.

[1] Buttocks.

Karezza the Beautifier

When the full magnetic rapport of Karezza has been realized, in which the two souls and bodies seem as one, supported and floating on some divine stream in Paradise, all sense of restraint and difficulty gone, and succeeded by a heavenly ease, power, exaltation, pure and perfect bliss, diffused throughout the entire being, it is then that the eyes and faces shine as though transfigured, every tone becomes music, every emotion poetry. And this normally continues for a long time, perhaps hours, gently subsiding, finally, into a sweet, contented lassitude and child-like slumber. But even to the last moment of consciousness there is a most clinging and tender affectionateness and desire to be close to the loved one, gratitude for the gift of such joy; nothing of that indifference or revulsion usually concluding the orgasmal embraces. And this continues after parting, even for days, so that one walks in a heavenly dream, and where the embrace is often repeated, tends to become a fixed and continuous habit, resulting in the most ideal love; if the parting is permanent, remaining in the memory for years, causing ever a gentle and tender reminiscence to pervade the thought of the loved one.

It is because of this that Karezza, though a sex act, so wonderfully increases and makes enduring the heart love. It is the embrace of the angels; sex sublimed by soul.

And because of all this it excels all other forces or influences as a beautifier. The faces of those who practice it tend to become exceedingly beautiful, on the spiritual plane especially; that is to say, it is the beauty of expression that is developed, rather than that of feature, though the features surely but more slowly follow, a serene, sweet light in the eye, a delicacy and refinement of line, a radiance and play of feature, a glad timbre in the voice, that vibrates an inexpressible magnetism and makes even the plainest personality fascinating.

Owing to the blending of the two natures, their mutual exaltation and reception of each other's moral qualities, it is soon to be noted that lovers who practice Karezza display the fruits of such inspiration and transmutation. The woman becomes strong, proud, confident, logical - displaying the finer masculine - while the man becomes gentle, considerate, compassionate, sympathetic, intuitive — revealing the finer feminine. Thus the sexes spiritually change and interweave and become at-one.

Is it any wonder if this most vitalizing of all elixirs, thus habitually fed to them, should make the organs receiving it, or through which it passes, beautiful, magnetic, graceful, radiant with life? Look at the lips, eyes, cheeks of a happy bride and find your answer. Joy is the greatest beautifier on earth and there is no joy like sex-joy. I prophesy that when Karezza becomes the habit of the people, made easy and perfect by inheritance developing into instinct, that the human race will become beautiful exceedingly, beyond the beauty of all former times; a subtle, inward beauty, shining through. The sex-force, which produces such rapture when felt locally, such a divine ecstasy when diffused in Karezza, will be healing in the hands of the physician, eloquence on the lips of the orator, fire in the eyes of the leader, genius in the brain of the great.

The Danger of Excess

The accusation is continually brought against sex-reformers that they become "obsessed by sex" and rush into excess. And this is sometimes deserved, for the tendency to excess exists in every intense nature toward whatever activity may predominate in interest.

But it is no condemnation of any pursuit to prove that it may be indulged in to excess. Its merit or demerit must be shown quite aside from the behavior of its advocates. For excess manifests itself everywhere. Nothing can be imagined more innocent than useful labor, intellectual study, or the desire for safety, yet every day we observe men ruined by overwork, blind or neurasthenic [1] from over-study, or cowardly or weak from excess of caution. Most of the accusers of excess in sex are religious, yet excess in religion, leading to bigotry, fanaticism, religious insanity, is among the very commonest forms of abnormality. To seek physical perfection is certainly most praiseworthy, yet few athletes escape an overstrain in training or competition that damages or kills.

It is common to praise "love" in opposition to sex, but love, so far as it exists apart from sexual expression, is peculiarly prone to excessive manifestation. Maternal love is perhaps the typical and purest form, yet in almost every mother we see her love become over-indulgent, partial and blindly unjust. The jealousy almost always present in the deepest loves, no matter how spiritual, proves excess, and when love is denied or suddenly withdrawn, unhealthful, insane or criminal symptoms almost always supervene, requiring all the powers of the spirit to quell. With every virtue known to man the same is true. In proportion to the power of any faculty, or the richness and value of any emotion, is the peril of excess. And sex shares this danger with the rest.

The reproach of excess, in many cases, is the result of mere prejudice. There is still an immense amount of theological odium attached to sex in the popular mind. It is a thing apart, to be kept secret and mentioned with bated breath, a thing doubtful and suspicious, if not certainly vile. To those who think thus, all frank interest in and attention to sex is excessive. And there is another large class who have themselves only abnormal interest in sex, knowing it only from experience of lust. To them all interest in sex borders on debauch. A man who studies sex, or writes on sex, is sure to be denounced by such people as "obsessed by sex," yet there is no more reason why a sexologist should not devote himself to the study and elucidation of sexual phenomena, than there is why an astronomer should not study stars or a geologist rocks.

But as sex is interwoven with our deepest feelings, the fountainhead of some of our strongest emotions, it is certainly liable to excess and far be it from me to deny this. There is a very real peril that those who are very loving and strongly sexed may give too much of themselves to the absorbing concerns of passion. A due proportion and balance is necessary in everything.

It is perfectly true that the wine of sex may sometimes go to the head and lead to a preoccupation with sex bordering on satyriasis or nymphomania, just as any other passion may become an emotional intoxication. Love and sex are subject to the universal laws of excess and satiation. Love and the thrill of sex are delightful feelings and we strive to hold them and intensify - this is natural and right within reason, but if continued too long the inevitable result is that the nerves become powerless to appreciate or respond. We may drain the reserves of the other faculties by diverting them all to sex - may thus indirectly weaken and atrophy them and finally may end by devitalizing love and sex themselves. And lovers are prone to spend time and money lavishly on their delight and may thus waste. Loss of sleep is a common source of love-waste too little considered. And in the man there are often the crude losses of the orgasm. There may be a feverish state of the system developed in which appetite and digestion are impaired and application or effective work become impossible; or an abnormal loneliness, destroying appreciation of or contentment with the usual joys of life.

Uxoriousness, [2] or slavish devotion and idolatrous admiration, may cause one partner to abdicate vindication of selfhood and spoil the beloved.

Those who are weak or moderately developed in sex may be less in danger, nevertheless it is to be remembered that the weak person may be overdone by an amount of expression that would be nothing to a stronger one. Excess is an individual matter which each should observe from the center of his own personality.

Those who practice Karezza are less liable to excess, because spared the waste of the orgasm, and because in them the emotion is sublimated and diffused, including soul, body and mind, the entire selfhood, yet they also may overdo. Excess here is more apt to manifest itself in the form of exhaustion from loss of sleep, or from too prolonged stress of tender emotion, or perhaps merely in the form of diverting too much time from other interests, rightfully precedent. There are cases too, not well understood as yet, in which one party exhausts or demagnetizes the other, perhaps acts consciously or unconsciously as a vampire, or in which both mutually exhaust each other.

Such symptoms are sometimes observed by two people merely in each other's presence, with no reference to sex, and are not necessarily coincident with any excess, but belong rather to the department of mal-adjustments and misfits, yet may unfortunately co-exist with a good deal of the finest mutual love.

It is possible to embrace too frequently in Karezza, or maintain the embraces too long. Only experience can determine what is moderation and what excess.

Those who do not use Karezza are vastly more liable to excess, and this usually from too frequent and intense orgasms, too frequent pregnancies, or too coarse, cynical and invasive an attitude. Where there is merely a physical itch or craving gratified, with no mutual tenderness or kindness, or perhaps actually against the desire or protest of one party, sex is always excessive.

If there is no indulgence except where there is mutual consent and enjoyment, mutual kindness and consideration, careful regard for the conditions of health and useful living, and a dominant conviction that all physical acts should express beauty of soul, there need be no fear. Excess is only where the act is individually or socially detrimental.

[1] [suffering a nervous breakdown]
[2] [foolish fondness for, or excessive submissiveness to, one's wife]

Final Considerations

It will be noticed that I lay great stress upon the value of love in Karezza and of refined feeling. For success there cannot be too much of both. Great love and poetry of feeling represent the ideal in the practice of the art of love. But I never forget the limitations of real life. Not all people can be poets. And I quite recognize that it often happens that very good people wish to marry or unite their lives, because they are lonely or physically starving, who yet have not and never could have any great, mutual romantic love. The practical question is: Can such successfully or beneficially practice Karezza? Certainly. The mere skeleton or essential framework of Karezza is this: That the parties be honest and kind toward each other, sexually healthy, the woman willing, the man potent, mutually at peace in their consciences about the matter, and united in their desire that there shall be no orgasm on the man's part. On this basis they can succeed and with benefit, but their happiness and peace will be very inferior compared to what it would be if deeper and higher emotions could be included. But when two pure and trustful friends once begin a relation of this kind, it seldom fails to go on to more beautiful attainments. Karezza seems to create inevitably a tendency to caress and be tender. It is a sort of natural marriage ceremony, which marries more and more with every repetition.

In relation to Karezza the question of the orgasm continually arises. The early writers on male continence, I believe, all argued that the seminal secretion resembled that of the tears, was normally secreted and reabsorbed and need never be discharged, except for procreation. Other physiologists, of a later date, declared that the semen, once secreted, could never be reabsorbed and must find discharge, thus denying those who have contended that reabsorbed semen was what gave the "illusion," the thrill, the virile feeling, the strongly sexed man knows. It is now believed that this inspiring elixir comes from the ductless glands.

It is very well to have a healthy scepticism about science as about theology. The theories and assertions of science too often crumble and fade before our very eyes. What we *know* from experience and observation in practice is a safer guide. And the practical facts are these: An accumulation of semen does occur in almost every man, sometimes, varying very much with different men, which apparently must have vent. It is a surplus. Either more has been secreted than can be absorbed, or, once secreted, it cannot be absorbed. Anyway it will come out. In the man who has nothing to do with women this causes the "wet dream," which is a perfectly natural way of getting rid of a surplus. In Karezza it causes the occasional failure. At least it is one cause. For no matter how expert the Karezza artist, the occasional failure to restrain the orgasm must be counted on. That beautiful equilibrium between the parties which leaves both so satisfied sometimes fails to occur and the man's orgasm irresistibly approaches, he is obliged to withdraw, and his Karezza becomes a *coitus interruptus.* The success of Karezza appears to depend on the sublimation of mere sex feelings into predominance of love feelings, and upon a diffusion of sex-consciousness so that too much is not concentrated locally. If local concentration becomes too great, an explosion inevitably follows. I have observed that if the woman a man loves becomes suddenly cold or angry toward him this local concentration is very apt to occur. It is more apt to occur with a fickle and moody or coquettish woman than with a steady and deep one; with a weak woman whose passion is fitful than with a strong woman whose great passion lifts and carries her partner on an even tide. It is harder to be continent on a full meal than on an empty stomach; harder soon after a bath. A vivid emotional experience of any kind may cause it, or intense intellectual exercise. The approach of a change in the weather, if sharp and marked, especially a "cold snap," may bring it about. It is all right and not to be worried over. *Coitus interruptus* used to be considered very bad for the man, but the modern view is that it is harmless, but may affect the woman nervously by leaving her unsatisfied. But this does not apply to the well-trained Karezza couple because, first the woman has the relation so frequently and so satisfyingly that she can well afford an occasional lapse; and, secondly, she knows that in a few hours, perhaps in a single hour, she may have it again, usually rather better than ordinarily, therefore has no excuse for nervousness. Just as the man must always be kind to the woman and stop the relation at any moment if she grows weary, or for any other reason wishes it, so the woman must be kind to him, cheerful, sweet and patient if he sometimes fails, and by this calling up of her affectional nature effectually cures the morbid self-pity which might make her nervously ill. Most men feel that they must have the orgasm at certain intervals, and there are scientists who have claimed to have discovered a sexual rhythm or periodicity in man which would seem to support this. But this sexual cycle in man appears to occur from once in four day to once a month, according to the individual. On the other hand almost all women want intercourse very frequently and long and leisurely each time, and sexual scientists support this too. It is admitted also by the highest authorities (they do not know Karezza) that *coitus interruptus* is the surest of all ways to avoid undesired pregnancy, while the contraceptives are none of them safe. Now all these things can be reconciled in Karezza. Let the man learn Karezza and his wife can have intercourse as often and as long as she likes, while the occasional failure gives him the relief of the orgasm at the time of his "period" or some other time.

And there is the question of the woman's orgasm. It is held by quite a good many men, some women, and many physicians say the same, that a woman also needs the orgasm, and that if she does not have it her health suffers. It is also commonly claimed that the woman's orgasm is essential in conception for the best results.

With these contentions I disagree. I consider the female orgasm an acquired habit and not natural. The male needs the orgasm to expel the sperm, but the female has no analogous need - her orgasm has nothing to do with expelling the ovum.

In all the animal embraces I have been able to witness, while the orgasm of the male was evident, I could see no evidence of a female orgasm. If the female orgasm is not necessary and does not occur below woman, why should it be necessary of occur *in woman*?

"To give her pleasure," is the answer, and a good one, but I hold that if she will have Karezza, she can have a finer, sweeter pleasure without it.

My objections to the female orgasm in Karezza (for it is to be noted that in the original "male continence" the woman had the orgasm if she wanted it) are threefold:

That self-control is more difficult for the man where the woman thus indulges herself.

That after her orgasm the woman is less magnetic, enthused and delightful as a partner, enjoys the Karezza less, and quite often soon becomes indifferent, depressed or irritable.

That indulgence in the orgasm on either side cultivates the merely sexual at the expense of the affectional, the romantic, the spiritual.

As I know that a woman who has known the perfect orgasm may deliberately abandon its practice completely in favor of Karezza, on the ground of its being less satisfying than Karezza minus all orgasm, and as I know that women who have never in all their lives had an orgasm may be beautifully satisfied and blissfully happy as well as healthy in Karezza without it, and this more and more as the years go on, I feel that I have good grounds for saying that I believe the orgasm in the woman is entirely unnecessary and artificial and that she is better off without it.

The ordinary male orgasmal embrace seldom satisfies the woman. It is too brief and animal for her. And if she is not satisfied in sex of course she suffers. But if she can have the orgasm with it, that gives her a kind of satisfaction, and that is why the orgasm seems beneficial to her, and her physician seeing the benefit endorses the act. But the same woman could be better satisfied in the non-orgasmal embrace of perfect and prolonged Karezza, and then the orgasm would be seen to be needless - that is *my* position.

My objections to the female orgasm in conception are as follows:

When a woman has an orgasm she has a discharge of vital-force and is left demagnetized, as a man is after an orgasm. I believe she demagnetizes the germ in so doing and that in this state it is less fit for impregnation than if there had been no orgasm - but this may be mere theory.

I believe, too, that the ideal way in the *procreative* embrace is for the man to waive all attempt at pleasure or to prolong the embrace, but to have his orgasm as quickly and forcefully as possible, directing all his magnetism into the seed and drawing nothing of her vital-force from the woman, but leaving it all for the child, and then to come immediately away and entirely withdraw from the room. The woman to have no orgasm, and to remain after the act quiet and recumbent for an hour or more. This also is theory, but at least I can say that where *my* advice was asked and followed pregnancy occurred, where before was sterility.

And this I *know*, that a woman can conceive without herself having an orgasm. There is every probability, I would say, considering the sexual lives of the average, that the majority of women conceive without it. I believe she conceives more easily and surely without it, for it is reasonable to infer that the spasmodic motions and abdominal contractions of the orgasm would tend to expel the sperm and then leave the parts negative and flaccid, instead of avid and receptive.

I know that a woman can have conception without having an orgasm, have a normal pregnancy and easy parturition, give birth to a perfect child, destined to grow up beautiful and healthy in body and a genius in mind. What more or better can any mother do? There remains the further question of Karezza in pregnancy: I feel sure the woman is better off in pregnancy without the usual orgasmal intercourse. It is liable on the man's part to be too violent and to cause her injury. And for the woman herself to have an orgasm might certainly bring a miscarriage. But on the other hand, I believe an occasional very gentle and quiet and tender Karezza (the man being careful of his weight) is most beneficial to the pregnant woman, and even to the unborn babe which is thus bathed in the magnetic aura and enfolded in the love of both its parents.

The woman feels it a very great comfort to have her husband's love embrace at such a time and often peculiarly longs for it. I have never seen or heard of any bad results from it and I recommend its considerate use.

The advantages of Karezza, as a love-act and otherwise, may be summed up as follows:

- It permits the embrace more frequently.
- It permits full penetration, contact and motion to the fullest extent, with no intervening substance whatever, thus completely satisfying woman's greatest sexual craving, which is for long continued, tender touch, as deep as possible, as long as possible.
- It gives the slower, more deliberate, more luxurious nature of the woman plenty of time to be fully aroused and fully satisfied.
- It satisfies her love-nature along with her sex-nature - which to her is the most important thing.
- It removes all fear of pregnancy, so that she feels safe.
- It requires no lotions, douches, greases, tampons, plugs, pessaries, drugs, syringes, skin-pockets, rubber bags, napkins, getting up in the cold, or any adjustments whatever - it leaves the poetry of the act not only intact, but intensifies it. Thus it satisfies the imagination, the craving for the ideal.

Because it cultivates self-control and requires the sublimation and transmutation of the merely sexual into the tender, the loving, the gentle, the romantic, its inevitable tendency is elevating, not degrading, to redeem and purify sex, not only to maintain its perfect natural innocence, but to add to it the chivalrous, the moral, the religious, in an ascending scale. Thus it satisfies the mind and soul.

It gives complete birth control. [1]

A general knowledge and use of it must certainly lift most of the odium which now attaches to everything sexual, thus increasing the respect for and appreciation of sex, its liberty and exercise, thereby automatically removing gradually the curse of social reproach.

Between the well-mated it leaves no sense of weakness or exhaustion, but one rather of sweet satisfaction, fullness of realization, peace, often a physical glow and mental glamour that lasts for days, as if some ethereal stimulant, or rather nutriment, had been received.

As this satisfaction is always normally combined with a grateful affectionateness and tender yearning toward the partner, it maintains, increases and makes habitual the union.

Where properly and successfully performed between the well-mated it gives the most absolute and perfect satisfaction without the orgasm.

Withdrawing the sexual electricity from the merely sex-organs, distributing it throughout the system and discharging it from every part toward the loved one, exchanging with that loved one, every part so used is electrified and vitalized and becomes more beautiful - Karezza is the greatest beautifier.

And this satisfaction, joy and perfected love inevitably react to increase the general physical health and mental vigor - Karezza maintains youth and is one of the best of the health exercises.

[1] [This is not true. It does, however, make conception less likely.]

Appendix

A school of physicians has arisen which claims the orgasm as a most important function, beneficial, and justifiably attained by artificial means if natural ones are not available, including with apparent approval, masturbation and the use of mechanical and chemical contraceptives.

The chief evil of this teaching appears to be that it is calculated to leave the reader of little experience with the idea that orgasms are practically harmless, that excess is unlikely, and that if no immediate bad results are noticed the practice may be indulged in to about the limit of desire.

To understand this problem we must consider the endocrine system.

In the organism there are ductless glands whose function is to deliver energy. These glands and the varying power of their function, I conceive to have a most intimate relation to the orgasm, its need and nature. Where these glands work excessively we may have a condition of almost or quite maniacal energy, quite upsetting the usual inhibitions; or, at the other extreme, where their action is deficient, we may have depressions, weakness, melancholy, cowardice, neurasthenia. Sexual love inspires the ductless glands to action, which is one reason why it is so healthful and joy-inspiring. To those who have deficient action of the ductless glands, sexual love becomes most beneficial, giving strength, courage, optimism, because it brings their action up to normal, or nearer to normal. But to a man who has excessive action of the ductless glands, sexual love, or sex-relations, may so increase this that a painful tension is created even a state of emotional intoxication or madness that may be insane.

All sexual crimes, rape, jealous murder, outrages of "Jack-the-Ripper" type, originate in this sexual insanity caused by excessive action of the energy glands - or that is my theory. On the other hand bashfulness, impotence, occur where the endocrine glands do not work strongly, or work fitfully, and give rise to melancholy and an "inferiority complex" before the adored one.

The relation to the orgasm is this: In the normal man, under usual conditions, it may be conceived that the semen secreted is all absorbed as fast as secreted, no surplus accumulates, no pressure is felt. There is a steady, normal output of energy from the ductless glands, neither excessive nor deficient. That the semen can be and is absorbed I think is satisfactorily proven by the numerous instances where men have been sterilized by accident, disease, or intentional operation in such a way that the testicles are left unharmed, but the semen is cut-off from its natural outlet. After being once secreted only two things are possible - either it must be absorbed or it will form a swelling. It does NOT form a swelling, therefore it certainly is absorbed.

And the orgasm is not essentially a discharge of semen, for it is possible for a man to have an orgasm with no discharge of semen, and women, who have no semen, can have orgasms as violently as any man. An orgasm is essentially a violent emotional discharge of energy or nervous force. Fits of rage, weeping, etc. are often truly orgasmal, and in many cases serve as substitutes for sexual orgasms, as in hysterics. Where the ductless glands are excited to more than usual activity, energy accumulates in the nerves and a demand is felt for its discharge. If the thoughts are then sexually excited there will be a demand for a sexual discharge, especially if the excitation has been of a sort to cause the energy to accumulate in the sexual centers, causing congestion. For wherever the nervous energy flows the blood flows also and remains congested unless the energy is discharged or withdrawn.

Now observers report very differently as to after effects of orgasms. Some "feel like a sick dog," or report dizziness, lassitude, weakness, dimness of vision, perhaps vomiting or fainting, while others only feel relaxed and soothed or declare energy and buoyancy increased. Some can endure only one orgasm at long intervals of perhaps a month or more; others glory in daily orgasms or even a number at one interview. Even the same individual often experiences a wide range in power or in good or bad effects. How explain these differences in the testimony of good witnesses? I think an understanding of the ductless glands explains all.

There are those in whom these glands work with more than usual power and if the energy thus received takes the direction of the genitals for an outlet, such a one feels a tremendous need of an orgasm, and, if he has it, he feels it relieves and benefits him, and if his glands are excited by the sexual embrace they may rush more energy into the vacuum, even an increased amount, making repetitions possible until the pressure is lowered. During this the contagion of his emotions may excite the glands of the woman and she also may have multiple orgasms, or may have them anyhow because of her own endocrine flow.

On the other hand a man in whom the flow of endocrines, or hormones, is only normal may feel quite spent after an orgasm, demagnetized, and must rest before a repetition. If his glandular flow is weak and a surplus only slowly accumulates, then, if he repeats too soon, he may spend not only his too scanty surplus, but may draw on his reserves to a degree that may cause uncomfortable or even alarming symptoms.

But *must* the nervous sexual surplus find an outlet through the orgasm? Yes, say the doctors of the orgasmal school, or health suffers. Here is where I differ. They recognize a *coitus completus*, a *coitus interruptus*, a *coitus reservatus*, and I would add a *coitus sublimatus*, which may also be a *coitus completus* in another way. I teach an embrace in which, in its perfect realization, there is a complete dissipation of congestion, complete discharge of nervous surplus, complete relief from tension and a complete satisfaction. An embrace peculiarly suited to the weak, because its action is to increase the function of their ductless glands and to make strongly sexed individuals out of those previously afraid of sex or feeling themselves sexual failures; and which can also completely satisfy the normally strong.

But where the technique of the orgasmal school is followed this embrace can hardly be realized, especially by those of powerful surplus. For everything in their technique tends to create a local congestion which must find relief in orgasm or distress follows. A "mutual, reciprocal, simultaneous friction" must certainly produce this result. I teach an alternation of friction, one positive while the other is passive, or else mutual quiet, magnetation and sublimation being the object. With them the whole matter is sexual and tends *downwards* to a sexual conclusion. With me the sexual magnetism is generated simply as a current on which to carry the love message, or by which to create the love light, all to be *sublimated upwards* to a romantic, poetic, spiritual conclusion, satisfying sex incidentally. They would concentrate the energy on the genitals and I would diffuse it from the genitals throughout the system, from the sexual to the affectional, from sex-desire to romance, tenderness, spiritual exaltation and love, affording, I contend, more complete satisfaction than an orgasm, especially to the refined.

And their method requires always the use of contraceptives, or else observance of times and seasons (all such safeguards being conceded by the best authorities unsafe and unreliable), while my method may be used at any time, with "nothing between," and all of Nature's romance of touch unrestrained, with the certainty that where no semen discharges no conception occurs.

One believes he has discovered what becomes of the semen in Karezza - that it leaks backward and comes out in the urine. But better authorities claim that leakage of semen only occurs in diseased conditions, and not at all from continence. I think where the sublimation and absorption are carried to the right degree there is no leakage, but I think it possible that it occurs where the excitement exceeds the sublimation.

I am willing to concede that where the intercourse is of such a nature as to cause a congestion that is not sublimated, or where sexual congestion occurs and sublimation and magnetation are not available, the orgasm may have a necessary place. Perhaps it must be admitted that everything has somewhere its use.

The idea that when once the usual amount of semen has been secreted, secretion largely or completely ceases, only enough being secreted usually to replace what is absorbed, and this even under frequent or habitual sexual excitement, is, I believe, probably correct, and agrees with my own understanding of the matter. But ever and anon, with the usual man, a surplus does accumulate, is not sublimated, and an orgasm occurs.

The question of whether the woman's orgasm is essential to the best conception seems to have a new sidelight thrown upon it by the discussion concerning birthmarks and prenatal influence.

If, as most modern physicians seem to agree, there is no truth in the old theory of prenatal influence; if the germplasm is something separate, of which the individual sex-partner is only a carrier, as a postman carries a letter, but with the message within which he has nothing to do, then it would appear that the woman's orgasm or nonorgasm has as little influence as any other prenatal factor. Just as it would not really matter, so far as the message in the letter was concerned, provided it was delivered, whether the postman was quiet and normal, or had an epileptic fit at the moment of delivery, so it would not matter what the woman, or the man either, did or did not do, provided the ovum and sperm-cell were safely gotten together. Their motives and emotional states, according to this theory, do not count. Which would explain how a woman could be impregnated by the semen from a syringe; or bear a normal child even if raped; or if in a drug-sleep.

Again it must not be forgotten that conception, scientifically speaking, is the penetration of the ovum by the sperm cell and their coalescing. This rarely, if ever, occurs at the moment when the carriers are having their orgasm, but sometime after, often hours or even days after, at the moment when the sperm cell reaches the waiting egg. How can the previous orgasm have any effect then to devitalize him?

The idea that a child begotten where the mother has an orgasm would be more passionate or robust than where the mother has none may have a core of truth. A robust woman would, all other things being equal, be more likely to have an orgasm than a more mental type. This robustness, or lack of it, would likely be an inheritable character transmittable to the child as a trait of the strain. In other words, the orgasm would be a *symptom* of the mother's robustness, which the child would be likely to inherit, but would be in no sense a cause of that robustness or its inheritance. If the sperm-cell could get to the ovum of that woman, no matter how quiet she might be, the result would be just the same as if she had the most intense orgasm - unless indeed the magnetic state of the parents could have an effect to vitalize or demagnetize the germs, which is also something the sceptical modem physician rejects. Also her orgasm, in many cases, would be a symptom of her being in "heat," *ripe* for impregnation, but no matter how ripe she might be, if she were slow, the man fast, she could easily be impregnated without her own orgasm, with exactly the same results to her child. Which accounts for the well-attested fact that many women have been impregnated by the mere spattering of semen within the lips of the vulva. Finally, as to whether she did or did not get the orgasm would depend upon how much she was excited, not upon her procreative power at the time - as it is certain that a sterile woman may have intense orgasms.

To get the sperm-cell of a healthy male to the ovum of a healthy female is the one important matter in conception, and how it is done, provided it is effectually done, seems of minor importance, perhaps of no importance at all.

To sum up: The orgasmal school is honest but mistaken. Its fault is that it is a doctrine of the strong, only for the strong. Just as a wealthy man may spend money recklessly for a while and still not be poor, so a man rich in thyroxin and adrenalin may spend recklessly in orgasms for a while and not seem any the worse. And the method, taught by the orgasmal school is such that it *creates* a demand, by congestion, for the orgasm, which must then occur or bad results follow. But for a weak man to follow their advice is very dangerous and courts a nervous breakdown, while my method builds him up. That orgasms are weakening is easily proven. Just as the way to get real facts about alcohol is to consult life-insurance companies, so to get facts about the orgasm go to the stockbreeder. Business has no sentiment or prejudice. Every stockbreeder will tell you that to permit a bull or stallion to serve too many or too often is to devitalize him.